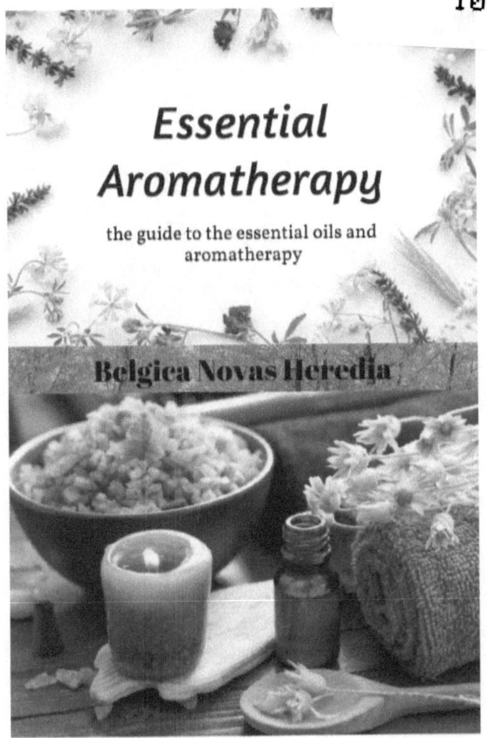

ESSENTIAL

AROMATHERAPY

ESSENTIAL AROMATHERAPY

the guide to the essential oils and aromatherapy

Belgica Novas Heredia

First to god because he is my guide in all the paths than i under-
take.
then to my children Bradley and Axel for being the best of my life

essential aromatherapy

A romatherapy has been considered down through the century as a remedy

that soothes the body and mind. The remedies are said to relieve

symptoms coming from a variety of diseases. In addition, the remedies

are claimed to relieve stress, anxiety, nervous tension, and related

symptoms. Many people have used aromatherapy, including the French

natives, Egyptians, Germans, Brazilians, Europeans, Indians, Canadians,

Americans, people in the Mediterranean lands, and so on. The oils

include the scented and essential oils. Online you can find a variety of the

oils, including Basil, Cedarwood, celery seed, carrot seed, African

Bluegrass oils, bergamot, clove bud and leaf oils, and so on. The oils each

have its purpose for healing the body and mind. Before using the oils be

sure to read all available instructions before using.

About Aromatherapy

Brief History:

Aromatherapy came from France, which a Frenchman burnt his arm,

dipped it in lavender oil, and concluded from the results that essential oils

and scented oils are healers. The result delivered ceased the burning, as

well there were no apparent scars on his arm. Essential oils and scented

oils are aromatherapy oils, which came from living plants. Exceptions

include the oils that came from swallowtail butterflies.

The intentions of the oils are to heal the body and mind by relaxing the

soul of stress. Few types of oils are intended to produce a romantic mood.

However, according to reports the best alternative for using aromatherapy

comes from massaging the oils into the flesh.

I've talked with a masseuse who claims that many of her clients

complained, since the oils made them feel drowsy, or put them to sleep.

Consequently, the oils must work to relax the body and mind; otherwise

the person would not feel drowsy or sleep when the oils are burn-ing. The

masseuse also mentioned that the green oils were prone to relax the body

and mind, more so than other scents. Now, whether this is true or not

would depend on the person and his or her level of stress.

As for aromatherapy creating romantic mood well the fact is down

through the years candle lit dinners, candle lit areas, etc have cre-ated a

romantic mood for many. So we can assume that aromatherapy can also

create a romantic mood. The romantic oils include Jasmine. Still, a

selection of aromatherapy oils can work as a romantic sparker.
Understand that aromatherapy romantic oils are essential oils. The oils

work to create synchronization with the spirit, mind, and body. The oils

are said to elevate moods through feeling by producing relaxation affects.

The affects are said to enhance well-being, confidence, and openness.

According to studies, few people using essential oils experienced a

hormonal affect, which increased desire of sexuality.

The oils available to promote romance are the Patchouli oils, YLANG

YLANG oils, Sandalwood, Jasmine, etc. The oils are said to deliver a

strong arousing feeling. The oils work by sending odors that stimulate the

moods and mind, which in turn produces an arousing sensation, as well as

an awakening yearning. Aromatherapy oils with aphrodisiac ingredients

are also romantic arousers. YLANG, Lemon oils, Patchouli, Rosewood,

Eucalyptus, Geranium, and Rosemary are a few of aromatherapy oils,

which contain aphrodisiac. Aphrodisiac Sensual oils are oil that produces

a romantic mood.

How do I choose oils for massaging?

Distilled oils, which are made from low temperatures and pressure, as

well as 100% natural graded A, oils is ideal for romantic massages.

According to reviews however, you should dilute the oils in the carrier

oil. Carrier oils is said to affect the skin, which produces relaxation.

Additional oils include the romance oils. The oils contain cedar wood,

clove buds, cinnamon leaf, clary sage, orange, and chamomile.

Yohimbe oils which include the Combinations work by increasing

erectile capabilities, libido, and sex
drives.

How do I choose the types of oils for different occasions?
You should learn more about the scents and essential oils to make your

choice. Lavender oils work to balance, elucidate, soothe, and regularize

the body and mind. Eucalyptus oils work to purify, cool, balance, and

revitalize the body and mind. Peppermint oils invigorate, refresh, cool,

and promote energy whereas Rosemary revitalizes, warms, and clarifies

the body and mind. Sweet Orange oils uplift your body and mind, as well

as produce a cheerful and stimulating feeling. Geranium lifts, balance,

stabilizes and relaxes the body and mind. Bergamot oils lift your moods,

normalize your mind, and build your confidence.

Aromatherapy Extracted to Heal

Aromatherapy works to heal the mind and body. The natural herbs, oils,

fragrances, etc aid in healing a wide array of diseases. At most

aromatherapy reduces irritating symptoms, as well as emotional

negativity's. Aromatherapy is used to heal the mind by relieving stress.

Down through the century's aromatherapy has been used by a wide

selection of professionals and individuals alike. India natives, Egyptians,

Germans, Frenchmen, Europeans, Brazilians, etc, have all used and still

use aromatherapy oils. After ongoing studies, research, etc, the oils has

proven to assist in promoting health. In fact, medical doctors use

aromatherapy in medical treatment. On the market is a variety of

aromatherapy scented and essential oils. The oils include asafoetida,

Cajuput, Celery Seed, Jasmine, Black Currant Seed, Carrot Seed,

Bergamot, Basil, and so on. Absinthe, Ajowan, African Bluegrass, Anise

Star, Anethi, Australian Balm Mint Bush, Arborvitae Wild are a variety

of other oils available on the market.

Australian Balm Latin name is Prostandthera Melissifolia. The flowery

plant was extracted through steam process. The oils origin is Australia,

which its flowers is shaped similar to a purple bell. The oils are pale

yellow once extracted, and works as an anti-bacterial agent. The oils

work as anti-fungal agents as well. Australian Balm will help reduce

colic, headaches, and colds. The medium scented oil blends with

peppermint, lavender, lemongrass, spearmint, and citronella. The oils are

non-toxic and are used as a cooking ingredient as well.

Ajowan is an essential oil, which its Latin name is Trachyspermum

Copticum. The herbs were extracted through a steam distillation process.

The origin of ajowan starts in India. Ajowan produces pale, yellowish

brown oils. The oils are essential for stimulating, and are used as anti-

spasmodic agents. In addition, ajowan has microbial agents, and

properties that help to fight colic symptoms. The strong scent blends with

sage, thyme, and parsley.

Ajowan is sometimes called Bishop Weed. The oils originated in India,

yet they are widely used in Egypt, Iran, Afghanistan, and Pakistan. You

must dilute the oils before applying to the skin, otherwise it could cause

irritation. If you're pregnant it is recommended that you do not use the

oils.

Anise Star in Latin is called Illicium Verum. The oils are extracted

through steam distillation process, and come from plant seeds. In

addition, Anise Star originates in China, yet it has a well-known usage in

various lands. Anise is a plant that grows licorice flavored seeds. The

Mediterranean plants are used in medicines, and to flavor drink and

foods. The Latin name is Pimpinella Anisum. The oils are clear, or light

yellow. Moreover, the oils are used to treat colic, rheumatism, and are

used in cough syrups, as well as pastille. The light scented oils blend with

orange, lavender, pine, clove, cinnamon, and rosewood. The oil is used in various lands as well as a breath freshener and aid to clear up the digestive system.

Arborvitae Wild is an essential oil, which its botanic name is Thuja

OCCIDENTALIS. The extraction of the needle and twigs from plants

occurred through a steam distillation process. The origin of these plants is
Canada. Arborvitae Wild is a confer tree, which is akin to the cypress

family. The flat leaves fit closely, which the leaves resemble scales.

The oils are pale yellow, which the oil is used as an anti-rheumatic agent,

anti-infection solution, anti-allergenic aid, etc. The oil is also used as an

insect repellent. In addition, you can use this oil as an anti-inflammatory

agent, to treat poison ivy, as an anti-microbial agent, etc. The strong

scented oils blend with cinnamon Bark, birch sweet, eucalyptus,

Cedarwood, cajuput, and cassia oils. Arborvitae Wild is considered the

oils of from the trees of life. The oils were used to ward off lightning.

Arborvitae Wild oils are to be used as instructed. We can now learn how

to use aromatherapy.
How to use Aromatherapy

While aromatherapy is made up of natural ingredients, it is smart to use

the remedies as recommended. Some of the essential oils can cause

nausea, vomiting, skin irritation, etc. Since we have a variety of articles

available discussing aromatherapy oils and how they work, I thought we

could switch up and learn how to use aromatherapy. Absinthe is one of

the essential oils available.

How to use Absinthe:

You should use absinthe oils as instructed. The oils include cautions,

which recommend that you do not use absinthe with aromatherapy

treatments. The oils have agents that work against aromatherapy, such as

neurotoxin, thujone, etc.

Absinthe is dark green oil, which is commonly used to treat anorexia. As

well, the oil is used to boost the digestive system, while promoting

menstruation. In addition, the oil is used to reduce fever, as well as

remove worms. The strong scents do not blend with other oils at this time. The prime use of absinthe was to eliminate tapeworms. A last word

of caution on absinthe is that people down through the years found that it

could be used as a drug for getting
high.

African Bluegrass is an essential oil. The oils can cause irritation to the

skin. You should also avoid using the oils around the eyes. African

Bluegrass is used as an astringent, anti-fungal agent, antiviral agent, and

is prepared and used to sooth the feet. The medium scent oils or strong

scent blend with floral and citrus
notes.
Angelica Root is another of the essential oils, which pregnant women

should avoid. The oils are non-toxic; however it is recommended that you

avoid using the oils in sunlight. The oil is commonly used in treating

gouty, arthritis, joint discomfort, congested skin, nervous tension,

migraines, bronchitis, fatigue, water retention, coughing, stress disorders,

and so on. The strong scents blend with sandalwood, Cedarwood,

Olibanum, and Guaiacwood.

Armoise Mugwort oils should be diluted before usage, since it is toxic oil.

The oils include neurotoxin and arbort-ifacient agents. Pregnant women

should avoid using this oil. The oil is used as an antispasmodic, and to

treat colic based symptoms. IN addition, the oil is used to discharge

worms, reduce stomach acids, and so on. The strong scented oil works

with oak moss, patchouli, pine, lavender, Rosemary, Clary Sage, sage,

Cedarwood, and so on. You can find this oil listed in Felon Herb lines as

well. St. Johns line may also have this oil listed.

Aromatherapy has a long line of essential and scented oils. Yet, each, oil

has its instructions, which you should follow to avoid harm. The oils are

intended to relieve the mind and body, which some oils are taking orally,

while others are not.

Bay essential oils is commonly used as an antiseptic, analgesic, antibiotic,

astringent, anti-neuralgic, insecticide, febrifuge, sedative, and so on. The

oils are claimed to treat colds, rheumatism, flu, muscle pain, skin

infections, dental infections, diarrhea, circulation irregularities, neuralgia,

and so on. The strong scented oil works with juniper, Cedarwood, ginger,

Ylang oils, geranium, coriander, lemon oils, eucalyptus, lavender,

Rosemary, rose, thyme, and orange flavored oils. Bay essential oils is

highly concentrated with Eugenol, which can irritate the flesh, mucus

membrane, and so on. It is recommended that the oils are used as

recommended and that pregnant women avoid using the oils.

A variety of other aromatherapy oils are available, including cardamom,

bergamot, caraway, bergamot-Bergaptene free oils, Cananga, Betal Leaf,

birch in both tar and sweet oils, cajuput, Cade, black currant seed oils,

Calamus root, Buchu, blood orange, Cabreuva, Camphor, Cypress

Australian Blue, Basil, and so on. Aromatherapy includes the essential

and scented oils.
Aromatherapy and Essential Oils

Scented Oils from Oils & Scents

Aromatherapy includes the scented oils. As well aromatherapy includes

the essential oils. The oils work by melting away your stress while the aroma fragrances relax the body, as well as the mind. Aromatherapy is

essentials and natural oils. The therapeutic oils allow you to utilize its

fragrances in a variety of ways. Aromatherapy oils soothe your body,

whilst spoiling the soft tissues of the body and relaxing the mind.

How to find aromatherapy scented and essential oils?

Online you can find a wide assortment of your favorite oils. The oils and

scents wash away the days stress. Aromatherapy is the choice which

helps you to relax. In addition, you can use aromatherapy oils to set a

romantic mood. The oils create a loving feeling, which each of your will

experience. In summary, aromatherapy will provide you a relaxing

moment in a romantic setting. Oils are also handy for decorating

warmers, or mists, since aromatherapy oils fill your environment with

natural and fresh scents.

Scented and Essential Oils create a peaceful environment. Aromatherapy

scented oils also works to enhance moods in your home environment.

Scented oils naturally generate sensual and loving moods, as well as a

feeling of relaxation. In fact, many masseuses' will employ aromatherapy

combined with reflexology, manipulation massages, and so on. The oils

help to relax the body and mind, while setting the
mood.

Which oils should I choose for romantic evenings?
IF you want to set the mood for both you and your partner, thus Jasmine

is the ultimate aromatherapy. Jasmine includes the Queen oils, which is

aromatherapy's essential oils. The scented aromas will set the mood, by

producing a luxurious scent. The scent works to create a loving bond

between you and your mate. The uninhibited aromatherapy oil is

irresistible and will put you and your partner both in the
mood.

Aromatherapy oils produce scents which surround your environment. The

scented oils will appeal to moods, memory, appetite, body, mind, etc.

You've almost certainly took notice of the advertisements, which

informed you of exotic, aromatherapy, scented, or essential oils.

However, aromatherapy, oils are natural oils, which differ from other

types of oils. Aromatherapy comes in a variety of scents, including

"Jasmine, Cedar, Lilac, Tuberose, and Myrrh. You have options however,

since can purchase a variety of natural scents, such as the enthralling

natural forest oils and floral scents.

Those feeling cheerful may benefit from the warmth of fig oils. The oils

will keep you in your cheerful mood. The warmth of fig oils includes the

orange and cinnamon scents.

The aromatherapy scents set the natural feeling or moods. You merely

smell the oils. In addition, the oils will supply new age solutions, since

you can use aromatherapy as air fresheners.

Why should I choose Aromatherapy over common oils?

Common oils incorporate chemicals, which will affect the body. You will

perhaps experience sinus problems, or related problems using common oils. In addition, aromatherapy oils set the mood in a natural environment.

Aromatherapy oils produce sweet smells in the air. Still, the scents will
not affect your sinuses or skin. Moreover, you will not need to invest in
products sold at local stores, which the unnatural fresheners will only
freshening your home for a short
time.

Online you can find a wide assortment of aromatherapy oils. The oils
again include the essential oils, and scented oils. Make sure you
understand the difference, since each aromatherapy scented or essential
oils produce a different effect. For instance, few oils are designed to spark
romance, while other oils are designed to lift your
moods.
Aromatherapy Essential Oils and Scented Oils

Questions of the day

You've probably read scores of articles related to scent and essential oils,
which arrive from aromatherapy. Probably what you haven't read is
articles informing you how the vendors decide on which oils to purchase

for resell. Since, you may have not read such articles will consider

vendors. Why...because how vendors decide can also help you decide

which aromatherapy oils are right for
you.

How do vendors decide which scented and essential oils are best for

marketing?

Vendors typically consider flavor, medium utilized for sell, tar-geted

selections sold in society, purpose intended,
cost, etc.

Base idea:

Scented and essential oils, such as the aromatherapy oils work to melt

away daily stress. The fragrances work to relax the body and mind, which

provides a healing aid. Aromatherapy essential oils and scented oils are

organic oils that derived from living plants. The therapeutic oils make it

easy for you to take advantage of its scents in a variety of ways.

Aromatherapy scented and essential oils soothe the body and mind, at the

same time the oils pamper the skin. Vendors and purchasers choose their

favorite oils and designer fragrances based on the volume sold.

The

aromatherapy oils assist those with overwhelming stress, by relaxing the

mind and body. In addition, vendors look for the oils that put you
in a

romantic mood. Vendors and purchasers alike no what
people like.
In addition, vendors and purchasers tend to search for decorative
home

warmers or misted oils that fill the environment with fresh and
natural

fragrances. People tend to enjoy the great out-
doors.

How long have vendors sold aromatherapy
oils?

Scented and essential oils or fragrance have been utilized for 100
years in

one fashion or the other. The oils were utilized to keep a pleasing
odor in

our homes and/or our work environment. In addition, purchasers
use the

oils to freshen their vehicle. At one time the oils were available in

selective flavors. Nowadays however vendors and purchasers
alike can

choose from hundreds of flavors varying from apple to orange.
African

rain and Ylang-Ylang oils are also available. Chinese started using
the

oils whilst promoting the oils as energy enhancers. Indians enjoyed

aromatherapy oils, since the oils were praying tools that aiding in what

they believed their god would hear from special oils dipped in wax sticks,

which they called agarbatti. Thus, the Indians believed that the oils would

create a spiritual milieu. The special oil flavored candles are available

today which are used for aromatherapy, similar to what the Indians used.

How do vendors and purchasers test aromatherapy oils?

Vendors and purchasers alike tend to test and try the oils through free

offers and samples.

One of first and foremost things that vendors and purchasers consider

while buying scented or essential oils, apart from the fragrance is the

packages. Attractive packages present substandard quality oils, which the

products could sell more than the higher quality oils. Moreover pricing is

an essential process of the decision making. Vendors typically search in

the middle, lower-middle, and related sections, targeting society's favorites. The price and package then is a demand that must meet modest

requirements.

The oils do not have to be dressed in fancy package, yet the oils must

present some attraction. The demand for aromatherapy in society is based

on price driven and high volumes of oils sold. Thus vendors must meet

the demand of supplies sold and society's likings.

How do vendors determine the best way to market aromatherapy?

The average method vendors consider for marketing aromatherapy

products is to advertise where customers frequent. Local supermarkets,

all-needs stores, flyers, pharmacies, etc are just a few areas that customers

visit often. Vendors may also consider targeting the upper middle

sections, which they will promote the products, airing them on television

or in global and local newspapers. Vendors will also offer free samples in

high-fashioned stores. Since the stores tend to sell fashion accessories for

the upper middle class people, vendors assume that the fragrance will sell. The elite sections are another area where vendors promote

aromatherapy oils. Choosing aromatherapy essential and scented oils can

be problematic, if you do not understand what orals can do for you.

Aromatherapy Essential and Scented Oils

Aromatherapy includes scented oils and essentials oils. The oils work to

dissolve away pressure whilst the fragrances aid in relaxing the body and

mind. The aromatherapy essential oils are organic oils, which are

designed to restore or maintain overall health. The oils make it easy for

you to utilize its fragrance in a variety of ways. Aromatherapy oils work

to calm the body, whilst mollycoddling the soul. At the same time the oils

relax the psyche.

How do I find aromatherapy oils?

Online you can select from favorite oils. Designed scents are available to

drown out all your daily stress. Aromatherapy oils assist in help-ing you

relax. As well, aromatherapy oils are available to put you in a romantic

mood.

Scented oils can also be utilized to decorate your home, which will warm

the environment. The mists of the oils will fill the area with fresh and

natural odors.

About Aromatherapy Scented and Essential
Oils

Aromatherapy scented and essential oils create a peaceful and loving

atmosphere. The oils set the mood while reducing stress from today's

over consumed society. When you work all day you will enjoy a moment

of relaxation with aromatherapy. Aromatherapy scented oils and essential

oils can produce outstanding feelings, whilst enhancing your mood. The

scented oils unsurprisingly trigger the physical and tender feelings that a

person will express. The aromas set the
mood.

How do I choose oils that will set a romantic mood for my partner?

Your partner will enjoy a romantic evening with aromatherapies Jasmine

scents. Aromatherapies Jasmine is the emperor of essential oils.

Jasmines

scented aroma expresses a loving bond, which your mate will likely

enjoy. Jasmine is not reserved, and the oil is irresistible. The scent will

definitely allure your mate into your
arms.

Aromatherapy oils aroma spreads all about your home. The scented oil

will appeal to your mate's mood. As well, the oils will ignite the memory,

and wet the appetite, as well as the body and mind. Jasmine, as well as

other aromatherapy oils are like no other scented or essential oils on the

market. The scented and essential oils come in a variety of fragrances and

scents. Jasmine, Lilac, Cedar, Myrrh, Tuberose, Rosemary, floral scents,

carrier, Absinthe, AJOWAN, African Bluegrass, ANETHI, etc, are just to

name a few aromatherapy oils available to you. Angelica Root, Bay,

Basil, Anise Star, Australian Balm/Mint Bush, ASAFOETIDA, etc, are

other types of aromatherapy oils available on the
market.

How do I choose aromatherapy oils that make me want to feel

cheery

although I am happy?

If you are feeling in good spirits you can stay in the mood by considering

the warmth of fig, orange and cinnamon oils. The scented oils will

supply you with the natural feelings or moods merely by smelling the oils

aroma. The oils can also be utilized as air fresheners. Oils which
include

chemicals can affect the nasal. As well the chemical based oils can
affect

regions of the body. Thus, non-chemical based oils can make your
senses

express your moods organically.
Aromatherapy oils produce a sweet aroma, which circulates in
the air.

However, the oils will not influence your skin in a negative light.
In

addition, you will not have to invest in products sold in general

stockpiles, which refreshes the air artificially. Now you can refresh your

home naturally with aromatherapy
oils.

How do I choose healing aromatherapy
oils?

The aromatherapy botanical oils are ideal for healing. The oils are
steam

distilled and derive from tree barks. Cinnamon oils are one of aromatherapies scented and essential oils that is made of cinnamon tree

barks. The oils come from evergreen native lands, such as Vietnam and

China.
Aromatherapy Oils

Aromatherapy includes essential and scented oils, yet the variants come

from a variety of resources. Aromatherapy is used for healing the mind

and body. The essential and scented oils came from plant extracts, as well

as other sources. Through distillations the plants fluids were diluted into a

watery substance, which produced the
oils.

How do I find aromatherapy oils? You can find aromatherapy oils online,

which is the better choice. Online you will have a wider selection of oils,

resources, vendors, etc. In addition, you can find the oils at discounts,

sales, bargains, or even find coupons to save on aromatherapy oils. You

may also find aromatherapy in areas were massages are practiced, fashion

shops, supermarkets, department stores, etc. Pharmacies sometimes carry aromatherapy oils. The smaller drug stores may not have a wide

selection; still they may carry the
oils.

How do I choose aromatherapy oils that will relax the
mind?

Aromatherapy includes the home therapy, which branches off in
self

treatments, cosmetic usage, and perfumes. Clinical therapy includes the

Pharmacotherapy and the Pharmacology. Aromatherapy includes the

Aromachology, which are the oils you want to choose if you are
looking

for psychological relief. The oils are claimed to affect the brain

positively. The odors send smells, which somehow makes the
mind relax.

How do I choose the aromatherapy
oils?

To choose aromatherapy oils you must first understand the types
of oils.

For instance, essential oils are fragrance which was extracted
from the

living plants. The chief process is distillation, which produced
aromatherapy eucalyptus oils. As well, expression oils, such as
the

grapefruit arrived from aromatherapy distillation.

Another of aromatherapy oils, include the absolute line. The fragrances

are extracted from delicate tissues found in plants, and flowers. The oils

are processed through artificial fluids extraction and/or solvents. ROSE

scents are one of the absolute aromatherapy. The oils may also come

from scented butter, enfleurage pomade, concrete, etc.

The natural volatile compound oils, which arrived from living plants and

are intended to eliminate microorganisms, is known as PHYTONCIDE.

Terpene is a variant, which the oils are established from sulfuric

mixtures, as well as from fragrant oils. Living plants is the main source,

which ALLIUM, which is PHYTONCIDE have disagreeing smells.

Therefore, you are unlikely to find aromatherapy oils, such as this brand.

Watery hydrosol oils are distilled as well, which produced the rosewater

oils. The oils are generally made from chamomile and roses. Infusion

aromatherapy is a watery extract, which came from materials found in

plants. Chamomile is a variant of infusions. The carrier oils are based

from TRIAYLGLYCERIDE. TRIAYLGLYCERIDE is utilized to dilute

aromatherapy's essential oils. The oils are designed to treat the flesh, or

skin. Sweet Almond oils are a skin healing aromatherapy oil. Lavender

scents are good oils for treating burns, or healing the skin
as well.

How do I know if I am purchasing aromatherapy
oils?

Well, it is difficult to tell, since various essential oils fall along the line of

aromatherapy providing it produces an
odor.
What is aromatherapy oils actually intended to accomplish?

The oils are intended to accomplish healing. As well, aromatherapy was

created to relax the body and mind, produce romantic surroundings, etc.

How can I decide if aromatherapy truly
works?

You can decide by asking friends who've actually tried the oils. Reviews

are available online as well. Be careful with reviews however, since many

are produced by vendors themselves. Ultimately, you can spend a small fortune to try the oils. The oils come in essential oils and scented oils.

How was aromatherapy invented?

A Frenchman burnt his arm, and due to the shock of the burn he instantly

dipped his arm in lavender oils, which ceased the burning and healed the

arm without causing apparent scars. Asking questions to help you better

understanding aromatherapy essential and scented oils:

Aromatherapy Questions

Questions of the day

You've probably read scores of articles related to scent and essential oils,

which arrive from aromatherapy. Probably what you haven't read is

articles informing you how the vendors decide on which oils to purchase

for resell. Since, you may have not read such articles will consider

vendors. Why...because how vendors decide can also help you decide

which aromatherapy oils are right for you.

How do vendors decide which scented and essential oils are best for

marketing?

Vendors typically consider flavor, medium utilized for sell, tar-geted

selections sold in society, purpose intended,
cost, etc.

Base idea:

Scented and essential oils, such as the aromatherapy oils work to melt

away daily stress. The fragrances work to relax the body and mind, which

provides a healing aid. Aromatherapy essential oils and scented oils are

organic oils that derived from living plants. The therapeutic oils make it

easy for you to take advantage of its scents in a variety of ways.

Aromatherapy scented and essential oils soothe the body and mind, at the

same time the oils pamper the skin. Vendors and purchasers choose their

favorite oils and designer fragrances based on the volume sold. The

aromatherapy oils assist those with overwhelming stress, by re-laxing the

mind and body. In addition, vendors look for the oils that put you in a

romantic mood. Vendors and purchasers alike no what people like.
In addition, vendors and purchasers tend to search for decorative

home

warmers or misted oils that fill the environment with fresh and natural

fragrances. People tend to enjoy the great out-
doors.

How long have vendors sold aromatherapy oils?

Scented and essential oils or fragrance have been utilized for 100 years in

one fashion or the other. The oils were utilized to keep a pleasing odor in

our homes and/or our work environment. In addition, purchasers use the

oils to freshen their vehicle. At one time the oils were available in

selective flavors. Nowadays however vendors and purchasers alike can

choose from hundreds of flavors varying from apple to orange. African

rain and Ylang Ylang oils are also available. Chinese started using the

oils whilst promoting the oils as energy enhancers. Indians enjoyed

aromatherapy oils, since the oils were praying tools that aiding in what

they believed their god would hear from special oils dipped in wax sticks,

which they called agarbatti. Thus, the Indians believed that the oils would create a spiritual milieu. The special oil flavored candles are available

today which are used for aromatherapy, similar to what the Indians used.

How do vendors and purchasers test aromatherapy oils?

Vendors and purchasers alike tend to test and try the oils through free

offers and samples.

One of first and foremost things that vendors and purchasers consider

while buying scented or essential oils, apart from the fragrance is the

packages. Attractive packages present substandard quality oils, which the

products could sell more than the higher quality oils. Moreover pricing is
an essential process of the decision making. Vendors typically search in

the middle, lower-middle, and related sections, targeting society's

favorites. The price and package then is a demand that must meet modest

requirements.

The oils do not have to be dressed in fancy package, yet the oils must present some attraction. The demand for aromatherapy in society is based

on price driven and high volumes of oils sold. Thus vendors must meet

the demand of supplies sold and society's likings.

How do vendors determine the best way to market aromatherapy?

The average method vendors consider for marketing aromatherapy

products is to advertise where customers frequent. Local supermarkets,

all-needs stores, flyers, pharmacies, etc are just a few areas that customers

visit often. Vendors may also consider targeting the upper middle

sections, which they will promote the products, airing them on television

or in global and local newspapers. Vendors will also offer free samples in

high-fashioned stores. Since the stores tend to sell fashion accessories for

the upper middle class people, vendors assume that the fragrance will

sell. The elite sections are another area where vendors promote

aromatherapy oils.

Aromatherapy Scented Oils

Aromatherapy is essential and scented oils that work to melt away your stress. The oils fragrances help to relax the body and mind.

Aromatherapy's essential oils produce natural scents, which

therapeutically drown away your stress as you utilize the fragrances in

many ways. Essential and scented oils soothe the body, while refreshing

your soul.

Online you can choose your favorites, which are designed to wash away

your daily stress. The different oils work by assisting you in relaxation.

Otherwise, you can purchase aromatherapy oils, which will set a romantic

mood. The oils also work as décors or warmers. You can use the oils to

freshen and fill the environment with fresh natural
scents.

SCENTED OILS

Both fragrant and scented oils are available. The oils have been utilized

for centuries by natives. The oils in various lands work to produce

pleasant odors in homes, cars, and workplace. At one time you could only

purchase a selection of aromatherapy oils. However, today there are hundreds of scents, flavors, etc available to you. You can choose from

apple scents, orange, or from the African Rain scents. Yiang Yiang scents

are also available as well as Jasmine. Chinese people at one time utilized

aromatherapy, as well as promoted its scents as an energy flow

stimulator. Indians employed aromatherapy while praying to their gods.

The Indians used the oils in the form of unique oils dipped in wax sticks.

The sticks were known as AGARBATTI. Agarbatti was believed to

devise a spiritual habit that would produce
peace.

The oils are available today. You can find special flavored oils online.

The oils are used as aromatherapy. Still, the flavors, scents, etc, depend

on a variety of factors.

When considering aromatherapy oils, think of flavor, targeted sections of

society, cost, purpose, and the designs of the bottles sold. As well, you

want to consider the medium of usage, as well as the cost of sell-
ing them

if you intend to become an aromatherapy
vendor.

Online you can find aromatherapy websites. The sites may offer you free

samples, which you can try out. Having the option of trying aromatherapy

oils, puts you in the front seat of making a good decision when buying

scented or essential aromatherapy oils: One of the hugest decisions made

when buying aromatherapy scents, is apart from the packages, the smell

is the focus. Online you can locate attractive packages, which are inferior

quality oils. In addition, you will find packages online, which focuses on

giving you economical selections. If are searching for specifics, you may

want to look in a variety of sections. Many aromatherapy scents are

packed accordingly to the modern demands.

Where do I find aromatherapy scents?

You can find a wide assortment online. Otherwise, you may find

aromatherapy scents and flavors at your local supermarkets, department

stores, etc. Since, the demand for aromatherapy products is price-driven, as well as high volumes can be sold and supplied at many local areas, you

can find aromatherapy at many locations. The intermediate fitting for

purchasing aromatherapy products would be the local supermarkets and

all-needs stores, flyers etc. On the other hand, you may find aromatherapy

at exotic stores, fashion stores, and related areas.

How do I decide which oils are best suited for romantic occasions?

The Jasmine line has a wide assortment of aromatherapy scented and

essential oils. Few of the oils used in massage therapy include the

Almond Oils, and the Apricot Kernel oils. The oils work as relaxing

flavor. While you can use them in massage therapy, you can also use

them for romantic evenings. In addition, the Apricot Kernel Flavors

include vitamins, which work to reduce aging. Aromatherapy is a way to

live well.

Living Well with Aromatherapy

Aromatherapy is an alternative medicinal remedy, which is related to

CAM. (Complementary & Alternative Medicine) Aromatherapy is

made

up of liquid plants, or materials. Aromatherapy can be found in the

essential and scented oils area. The aromatic scented oils are another area

was you will find aromatherapy. The mixture of plants is said to have an

effect on health and moods.

Aromatherapy has been in existence for some time. The oils were quickly

put on the market after a French man discovered that the oils could heal

burns without scarring the flesh. He had suffered a dramatic burn while

working in his laboratory, which immediately he dipped his arm in

lavender oils. He got good results, which lead to aromatherapy and the

notion that it can heal the body and
mind.

Aromatherapy comprises a set of branches. The branches include

perfumes, self treatments, home therapy, cosmetic usage, clinical therapy,

pharmacology, pharmacotherapy, Aromacology, etc. Aromacology is the

process of healing the psyche by using odors and scents that affect the

mind.

Aromatherapy includes essential oils, which are fragrances that were

extracted from living plants. The extracting process produced

aromatherapy through distillations, which included eucalyptus oils.

Grapefruit oils were also produced through distillations of plants.

Aromatherapy also includes the absolute fragrances which were extracted

from delicate tissues found in plants, and flowers. Aromatherapy was

created from these sources through a solvent process or else an extraction

of artificial fluids. Rose fluids made up Rose Essential Oils in the

absolute category of aromatherapy. Rose Fragrances described the

extracted oils that arose from concrete, scented butter, ethanol, etc.

Aromatherapy includes the PHYTONCIDES. The organic volatile

compounds came from the roots of plants, which where utilized to

annihilate microorganisms, also known as microbes. The oils are based

from terpene, or sulfuric plant compounds. Terpene is the larger class of

diverse hydrocarbons. The carbons are produced in living plants, which includes the prime plant life, such as the conifer. Conifer is a cone

bearing tree. In addition, carbons may also arrive from insects. The prime

insects may include the swallowtail butterfly. Carbon is also a chief

constituent deriving from turpentine, and resin. Turpentine is the prime

source, where terpene got its name. Terpene then is a prime ingre-dient

found in essential oils. You can use essential oils to add flavor to

foodstuff, perfumes, aromatherapy,
etc.

In addition, hydrosol is a variant of aromatherapy. Hydrosol is a watery

incidental product, which was distilled in Rose water. This is the scented

oils you can find in aromatherapy lanes. Hydrosol limits itself to

CAMOMILES and Roses. The purpose of limitation is that hydro-sol is a

colloidal solvent, which particles are often suspended in water, and

sometimes the fragrance is un-friendly.

Aromatherapy also includes infusions. Infusion is another watery extract

deriving from living plants. Infusion often comes from CHAMO-MILE.

Aromatherapy includes Carrier oil. The oil is extracted from

TRIACYLGLYCERIDE, and is diluted and produced as essential oils.
Sweet Almond Oils is one of aromatherapy's oils, which came from

carrier oils. The oil is utilized to treat the skin.

How do I know if aromatherapy will work for me?

You don't. Most times people have to use a large volume of scents and

oils to produce good results, according to reviews. However, theorists

have made many claims related to aromatherapy. In addition, many have

tried the scented oils and essential oils, which the results led to

practitioners using the oils as an herbal solution, naturopath, medicinal

remedy for infections, healing aids, etc. According to reports, the oils

work best when massaged into the skin, since it will set in motion the

limbic system, as well as the emotional section. In addition, aromatherapy

was known to set in motion the thermal receptors. There is nothing like

relaxing with us we smells of aromatherapy.

Relaxing with Aromatherapy

Aromatherapy is natural oil, which helps you to relax. The oils are

distilled from natural plants, tree barks, swallowtail butterflies, etc.

Online you can find a wide assortment of aromatherapy oils, including

the essential oils and scented oils. The natural oils work in a several ways

to help you find relaxation. Still, you want to be careful when shopping

for aromatherapy oils, since the market is swamped with substitutes.

Since, scents, fragrances, essential oils stand out, aromatherapy oils are

now hard to define. Therefore you want to look for oils that come from

natural resources.

Essential and scented aromatherapy oils are either distilled from steam.

Rarely are the oils concentrated or produced from unnatural solvents.

How can I tell if the oil is aromatherapy based?

Well, I basically covered this question, however it is a good question still,

since some vendors will actually claim that the oils are from natural

sources when they are not. Therefore, we can consider aromatherapies

base, creation, types, etc, to help you avoid purchasing non-
aromatherapy

oils.

Carrier is one of aromatherapies oils. Yet, few vendors may dress carrier

up, disguising the oil as aromatherapy organic oil. To help you

understand carrier oils, please consider.

Aromatherapy is a treatment that works by producing natural fragrances

deriving from plants. The oils are extracted from living plants to alleviate
psychological and physical disorders. The oils usually work by inhaling

the oils, or through massage therapy.

Carrier oils are an oily plant, which its roots came from Triacy-
glyyceride.

The constituents are employed to dilute aromatherapy essential oils. Once

the substance is diluted it works to heal the
skin.

African bluegrass is botanical oils presented as an aromatherapy
essential

oil. The botanical aromatherapy name is listed under Cymbopogon

Validus. African oils were extracted from solid meadow tufts and
was

distilled under steam. The oils derived from South Africa and is
an

unrelenting, aromatic oils stemming from grayish green lands,
which

produced a lemony scent. The aromatic oil is light yellowish
in color.

Africa's bluegrass has a history of producing harsh, anti-fungal
remedies

in addition to its anti-viral production. Africa then uses African
Bluegrass

aromatherapy to treat the feet. The oils are thin and consist, yet
the

strength of its scents is medium or else
strong.

African bluegrass will blend with citrus scents. Soft flowery notes
will

also work with African bluegrass. The scent of the oil produces
sweet,

grassy, herbaceous base, i.e. similar to dills, sage, or thymes. The
oils are

fresh and light scented, yet smells organic.

African oils achieved its history from Cymbopogon. The name

came

from Greece kumbe, which defines pogon and/or nacelle. The terms mean

bore. Ancient history claims that the African bluegrass oils are arranged

with holy oils. The holy oils include citronella, olive, myrrh, and groove

oils. Apparently some people want to avoid this oil, since it can irritate

the skin.

One of the safer botanic oils along the line of aromatherapy is Vitis

Vinifera. The oils were developed from natural fruits and ex-tracted under

steam. Cognac as it is named derived from aromatherapies ori-ginal origin,

which was France. The cognac oils derived from natural fruits, such as

grapes. Since the grapes used also makeup few of the ingredients in

brandy, aromatherapy named the oils cognac. The oils are light yellow,

which some oils are green-yellowish. The oils are often employed to act

as perfumes or flavors. Cognac works as an after-shaving lotion or

cologne and presents an uplifting feeling from its organic fruit aroma.

You can also use cognac with tobacco correlated inventions. Cognac is consistent in thick and medium scents. Cognac has a strong aroma, which

it blends with galbanum oils, bergamot, all lavender oils, coriander, clary

sage, linalool, Ylang Ylang, etc. Aromatherapy is a aid that works like a

healer.

Aromatherapy Aiding as a Healer

Aromatherapy aids as a healer. A variety of essential oils and scented oils

are available online, in drugstores, fashion stores, etc...

Bergamot is one of the top aromatherapy aids. The aid works to relieve

stress, hysteria, fear, anxiety, fatigue, gouty, arthritis, bronchitis, water

retention, migraines, nervousness, jammed skin, etc. The sweet aroma is

strong solutions that aid in healing the soul and mind. Bergamot's variant

is the Bergaptene oils. The botanic oils are also referred as citrus

Bergamia. Bergaptene oils are extracted through cold press procedures,

and are extracted from rudimentary fruit peels. The oils derived from

Italy, yet is found in South East Asian lands, Europe, Tunisia, Morocco,

Ivory Coast, etc. Bergaptene comes from Bergamot, which is an

Asian

based spiny citrus tree. The tree grows sour pear-shaped fruits, and its

Latina name is Citrus Bergamia. Aromatherapy oils were extracted from

the fruits, which the fragrances are yellow-green and is listed in the

essential oil section. The fruits rind was used to make the oils, which

produced perfumes. Mediterranean mint plants are a source linking to

Bergamot. The fragrances are similar in comparison, and its Latin name

is Mentha Citrata.

The oils aid in healing. The common usage is to treat depression,

hysteria, fear, infections, anorexia, eczema, psoriasis, stress, anxiety, etc.

In summary, Bergaptene aids in healing. The aroma produces a medium

affect. You can blend this oil with Jasmine, Ylang, Geranium, Clary

Sage, Nutmeg, Mandarin, Cypress, Frankincense, Rosemary, Orange, and

Sandalwood. If you are searching for a sweet fruity smell, this is the oil of

choice.

Benzoin is aromatherapy essential oils known as Styrax Benzoin. Its

botanical oils, which arrives from resin. Resin is an organic substance,

which comes from plants. The plants are firm and secrete sap
from the

plants and tree. Resin has a yellow and/or brownish color.
Benzoin was

extracted from food grade solvents. In addition, benzoin originated from

Sumatra, yet Thailand, Java, etc, grows the trees as
well.

Benzoin aids as an antiseptic. The oils aid by producing anti-

inflammatory and anti-depressant solutions. Still, the oils are
used to

relieve flatulence, colic, alimentary canal, water retention, colds,
cough,

eczema, acne, arthritis, rheumatism, psoriasis, scared tissues,
mouth

ulcers, chilblain, muscle aches, rashes, stress, circulation, nervousness,

etc. You can combine benzoin oils with Coriander, Frankincense,

Bergamot, Petit-grain, Sandalwood, Rose, Myrrh, Lavender, Juniper,

Lemon, Orange, etc. The oils produce a warm, sweet aroma,
which smells

similar to vanilla.

Arborvitae Wild is a botanical essential oil. The oils are sometimes called

Thuja Occidentalis. Arborvitae oils were extracted from twigs and

needles through a steam distillation process. The plants were originated in

Canada. This particular aromatherapy brand is also known as the Tree of

Life. Arborvitae is a coniferous tree. The trees derive from the Cypress

family.

The leaves of the Arborvitae like the Cypress have flat fitted leaves,

which resemble scales. The oils aid as anti-infectious-rheumatic-

allergenic constituents. The constituents are used to reduce psoriasis and

related systems. The oils are also used as insect repellants, anti-microbial

solutions, anti-inflammatory remedies, etc. The oils will also soothe

itching and irritation from poison ivy. You can blend the oils with

Cajuput, Cedar woods, Eucalyptus, Cinnamon Bark, Cassia, Birch Sweet,

etc.

Various other aromatherapy oils are available as well. Carrot Seed Oils,

Cassia, a variety of Cedar Wood oils, Celery Seed, Clove Leaf, Clove

Bud, Chamomile German, Moroc, and Roman, etc are available to you.

Cinnamon Bark and leaf, as well as Chilly Seed, Citronella, Clary Sage,

Citronella Java, etc, are all available to you.

Coffee, Cognac, Copaiba Balsam, Cumin, Curry Leaf, is additional

aromatherapy healers on the market.

Aromatherapy Solutions

Aromatherapy is the latest solution that has interested many.

Aromatherapy has been in existence for thousands of years. The remedies

were used by the Romans, Greeks, Egyptians, France, Chinese, etc. Egypt

doctors tend to recommend that their patients use aromatherapy by adding

the fragrances to their bathes. In addition, massage aromatherapy was

also recommended. In fact, Egypt used aromatherapy in the embalmment

process of the deceased. Egyptians then used aromatherapy as an

alternative medicine that healed the ill and dead respectively.

At one time various other sources, such as the Hippocrates used

aromatherapy as medicines, which some were also recommended in

bathes. Massages were another recommended remedy. In fact, the

Hippocrates used aromatherapy as a treatment alongside fumes to

disinfect, or kill pests. See Athens Plagues to learn more about such

treatments.

Nowadays, aromatherapy comes in the modern formulas. Aromatherapy

took off again after a Frenchmen in the Chemistry industry burnt his arm,

which he dipped his arm in Lavender oils. The results produced good

fruits. That is the results reduced scaring and healed his burning

sensations. He then dubbed the oils as therapeutic aromatherapy

solutions. Essential oils came into focus at this time as well. (1930)

During the 30s event, the Frenchmen was inspired by the respond to

dipping his arm in lavender oils, that he decided to run tests on related

oils. He came up with the notion psychotherapeutic, rather the benefits

that aromatherapy oils could produce to treat the body and mind. During
the 1940s, (WWII) another Frenchmen who was a military doctor made

use of essential oils by using the oils as an antiseptic. (Read Rene

Maurice Gattefosse and Jean Valnet to find additional information related to the history of aromatherapy; also see information related to Madame

Marguerite Maury) This lady came up with the holistic notion, i.e. she

deemed aromatherapy as social, mental, physical, and treatment for the

ill. Lady Maury also recommended massage therapy while using the

essential oils.

How does aromatherapy heal?

Aromatherapy heals through its natural scented fragrances. The essential

oils submit powerful fragrances, aromas, etc, which the odors impact the

person smelling the fragrances. The results touch the body and mind.

Aromatherapy includes the strong, medium and mild scents. The stronger

scents are ideal for anyone who has difficulty smelling. In fact, experts in

the medical field found that those seeking mental health for depression

and obsessive anxiety lack the ability to smell. According to research and

experts in the medical sector, the fragrances produced by aromatherapy

targets areas of the nose, which is known as the cilia. The cilia target the limbic system. The limbic system is near the limbus. The two work in

harmony and affects the brain region, where out emotions, intellect,

moods, and memory is controlled.

According to studies, lavender oils help the brain waves flow smoothly,

which produces an increase in the alpha waves. The waves are seated at

the back region of the head. The waves help us to relax, which if

aromatherapy scents target this area, it could provide relaxing affects.

Jasmine is aromatherapy oil, which targets the beta waves. The waves are

located at the frontal lobes of the head. The waves work to help us stay

attuned, or alert to what goes on around us. Aromatherapies Jasmine

targets these waves, which means the solution could augment awareness.

Aromatherapy was tested in science labs. The scientists concluded that

essential oils incorporated prime chemicals that our body and mind

produce naturally. The chemicals discovered were ALDEHYDES,

Terpene, ester, and alcohol.

Alcohol is essential for killing bacteria buildup. Alcohol also stimulates

the mind, energizes the body, vitalizes our well-being, diuretic, and acts

as an antiviral solution. In fact, the pancreas alone produces more than 30

types of alcohol. The alcohol targets the metabolism. If you are searching

for alcohol-based aromatherapy checkout the line of aromatherapies

Ginger, Rose, Sandalwood, Rosewood oils, Patchouli, Peppermint, tea

tree, and myrtle oils. Find the cures for you in aromatherapy treatment.
Curing with Aromatherapy

Imagine the sweet smells of aroma coffee perking in the coffeemaker.

Each morning when you arise you smell those sweet aromas that perk

your nostril. Well know you can add to that smell by using

aromatherapies botanical COFFEA ARABICA, or coffee essential oils.

The aromas were extracted from coffee beans, or plants. The flavors

derived from Brazil. The coffee oils in aromatherapy provide you a smell

similar to what you experience from brewed coffee. You smell the aroma

and start to feel invigorating and
warm.

Coffee aromas are described as the earlier cultivations where as
the class
of coffee trees where grown often. The species included CAN-
EPHORA
and ARABICA, which are fine coffees. Coffee aromatherapy is dark
oils,
which the coffee oils when burned will deodorize the environment.
Coffee is found to be a great antioxidant. Coffee oils work to help
those
smelling the aromas reduce depressive symptoms. Coffee is also
found to
soothe respiratory complications, fevers, bee or bug stings,
nausea, etc.

Coffee oils is unlike other aromatherapy aromas in that the coffee
oils
work best alone. Typically you can find coffee aromas in medium
or
thick formulas. The strength of the aromas is typically medium
or strong
scents.

The history of coffee oils spaces out. While minimal information
is
available, the Islamic Monks once utilized coffee oils, especially
when

one monk found it hard to stay alert while praying. He spotted a man in a

field, which appeared gleeful and asked the man what was his

recommendation. The man recommended the aromatic smell of coffee,

coffee beans, or oils. The man bent on finding alertness took comfort in

coffee aromas, which sparked the entire congregation. Africans, Chinese,

Brazilians, Latino, Dutch, etc, including America all found it easier to

stay awake while consuming or smelling coffee beans. Coffee is an

Abyssinian name, which is called CAFFA.

Cyproil is another of the dark aromas. The botanical CYPERUS

SCARIOSUS oil came from flower parts, which were extracted via

steam. The oils come from Brazil, just as the coffee beans. Cyproil oils

are grassy oil, which aromatic floral scents circle the air. The oils are

light brown, or dark amber colored. Cyproil is commonly utilized as a

perfume, which includes soaps, incense sticks, etc. The oils work as well

as a repellant to ward off insects, as well as a healing medicine. Cyproil

oils include the spicy oils, wood, earth, etc. The oils will blend with other

aromatic oils, such as Clary Sage, Bergamot, Patchouli, and Labdanum.

This particular oil was also used in the India lands, which the purpose

was to reduce digestion complications.

Cade oils fall along the essential oil line. The oils are botanical Juniperus

Oxycedrus, which the oil is made from woods and distilled via steam.

The aromatic derived from France, which it too is darker colored oil.

Cade oils come from evergreen shrubs. Cade oils are extracted from the

heartwoods and braches where needled shrubs grow black
berries.

Cade oils are commonly used as a liniment or ointment. The oils treat

severe skin conditions, eczema, PRURIGO, parasitic, psoriasis,

ringworms, etc. In addition, the oils are used as disinfectants, antiseptics,

antimicrobial, anti-pruritus, vermifuge, analgesics, parasiti-
cides, etc. You

can find medium aromas which blend with Clove Bud, Thyme, Cedar

Wood, Labdanum, Rosemary, and Origanum. The odors produced by
Cade include tar aromas, smoke, dry, etc, the oils are non-toxic. The oils

were commonly used in areas of France; however Africa and Europe now

use the oils.

Online you can find a variety of aromatherapy oils. The oils include

Absinthe, Basil, African Bluegrass, Angelica Root, Arborvitae Wild, Bay,

Benzoin, Ajowan, Bergamot, Blood Orange, Anise Star, Cade, Betel

Leaf, Birch Sweet, etc. Are you reading to start your healing process with

aromatherapy?
Healing with Aromatherapy

Aromatherapy essential and scented oils are said to heal the soul and

mind. Online you can find a wide assortment of aromatherapy oils, which

the oils have its own, focus. The oils can work as relaxing agents, healers,

decorations, fresheners, romance sparkers,
etc.

The oils available include bergamot, absinthe, benzoin, African bluegrass,

bay, basil, anise star, Australian balm mint brush oils, anethi, ajowan,

asafoetida, angelica root, armoise mugwort, arborvitae wild, etc.

Bergamot includes the Bergaptene free oils. This is one of aromatherapies

most popular oils.

Bergamot is botanical oil, which its Latin name is technically known as

Citrus Bergamia. The oils can from plant materials, which include Crude

Fruit Peels. The method of extraction is through the cold press procedure.

Bergamot's origin is Italy. The oil comes from tree plants, which the trees

flowers are shaped like a star. The leaves are smooth; as well the trees

bear fruit, such as citrus fruits. In addition, the tree resembles a grapefruit

and orange respectively, yet it is shaped like a pear. When the fruits are

ripe they are often are green at first and turn yellow. Actually, bergamot

is a spiny Asian citrus producing tree, which bores sour pear-shaped

fruits. The Mediterranean Mint plants are a variant of bergamot, which

the plants source is fragrant oils similar to the bergamot oils. The Latin

name for the Mediterranean plants is Mentha Citrata.

How do I know what bergamot oils are used for?

The oils are used as essential oils. The oils typically are utilized to treat depression, relieve tension and stress, etc. The oils have also helped in

relieving hysteria, fear, and related systems. In addition, bergamot works

to relieve infections. Those with eczema, general convalescence,

psoriasis, and anorexia can also benefit from Bergamot oils.

Bergamot is light oils, which its strength is typically medium. The oils

blend best with Clary Sage, Black Pepper, Jasmine, Nutmeg, Cypress,

Rosemary, Mandarin, Orange, and Geranium, Ylang Ylang,

Frankincense, Sandalwood and Vetiver oils. The oils named are common

aromatherapy oils marketed and sold at high volumes. The scent of

bergamot oils presents citrus, fruity, sweet, and balmy-peppery, flowery

aromas. Its evocative aroma mates with Lavender and Neroli oils as well.

Brief Bergamot history:

Bergamot oils first product was sold in Bergamo, Lombardy where it

originated. You can find bergamot trees in Lombardy, South Eastern

Asia, Europe, Italy, Ivory Coast, Algeria, Tunisia, and in Morocco.

How do I use bergamot oils?

You want to read the instructions carefully, since bergamot is highly

concentrated with Bergaptene, it has been known to cause severe burns.

This is especially true when the oils are used on sensitive skin.

Aromatherapy works that is best to heal
you:
Aromatherapy at its Best

Aromatherapy, at its best works to heal the body and mind, heal-ing it

from various illnesses, as well as working as a stress reliever to prevent

illness:

Aromatherapy has been used over the years by Egyptians, In-dians,

Europeans, Germans, France, etc. The oils have proven to assist in

relaxing the body and mind, and were used as a medicinal rem-edy.

Asafoetida is one of aromatherapy's essential oils. The oil's bo-tanic name

is referred as Ferula Assafoetida. The oils were extracted through a steam

distillation process, which came from the roots and stems of plants. Iran

is where the tree originates. Asafoetida is a recurrent native tree, which

Palestinians, Afghanistan, and Iran natives make use of the trees roots

and stems. Asafoetida is a strong smelly plant, which when extracted and

cooked presents a bitter, brownish and acrid smell. The Indians used the

oils while cooking meals. Asafetida plants are a sister to the parsley

family, which is where Asafetida is extracted. The Latin name is Ferula

Assafoetida.

Asafetida oils are used to relieve nervous disorders, muscle spasms, colic,

coughing, bronchitis, pneumonia, etc. The oils are also used to remove

parasites in the intestinal, including worms. In addition, asafetida oils

assist in relieving chronic fatigue, digestive sensitivity, candidiasis, etc.

The oils have a strong scent. In addition, the oils blend with onion,

cardamom, garlic, caraway, basil, and bay scents. Asafetida over the

centuries achieved a variety of AKA names. The Devils Dung, as well as

the Foods of the God was a couple of AKA's Asafetida is known for.

This oil is an ingredient of Worcestershire Sauce, and has no toxic agents

in its ingredients. It is recommended that you avoid using

Asafetida oils
while pregnant.

Cajeput is aromatherapy's essential oils. The botanic name is
MELALEUCA CAJEPUTI. The oils were extracted through the steam
distillation process and come from the leaves and twigs of plants. The
plant originates in Indonesia. The plant is a smaller
tree.

Cajeput is used to heal skin disease, urinary dysfunctions, intestinal, and
pulmonary problems. As well the oils are used to stimulate phlegm. You
can use Cajeput oils as an antiseptic, anti-neuralgic, analgesic,
antispasmodic aid, antimicrobial, carminative, insecticide, tonic,
febrifuge, diaphoretic, etc.

You can find Cajeput in medium flavors, which blends with Thyme,
Clove Bud, Rosemary, Cedar Wood, Labdanum flavors, Origanum, etc.
The White Tea Tree or Cajeput also is known as Paper Bark Tea Tree,
Broad Leave Tea Tree, White Wood, Swamp Tea Tree, etc. Again,
pregnant women are recommended to avoid using
this oil.

Celery Seed Essential Oils is a botanic APIUM GRAVOLEN. The oils

were extracted via the steam distillation process from plant seeds. The oil

originally comes from India. This pale yellowish oil is used as an anti-

oxidative. As well, the oils are used as an aid to treat rheumatic

symptoms, and are used as an antiseptic. The antiseptic aids in treating

urinary problems. The oils are also an antispasmodic remedy, aperitif, etc.

You can use the oils as a depurative, to heal the digestive system,

sedative, stimulate of the uterine,
etc.
The oils are also made up of detergents, soaps, perfumes, and cosmetics.

It is also used as flavors in beverages, and foods. The medium strength

remedy blends with pine, tea tree, lavender, spicy oils, LOYAGE, oak

moss, OPOPANAX, etc. The oils are frequently used in various parts of

the land, including Holland, India, China, the USA, Hungary, etc.

Pregnant women should avoid usage of this
oil.

Online you can find a wide assortment of aromatherapy oils, including

the essential and scented oils. The oils were designed with intents, which you will find helpful information online. In summary, aroma-therapy is

always an action to heal the soul.
Aromatherapy in Action

Aromatherapy oils include Bergamot, Bergaptene Free, Carrot Seed,

Cardamom, Betal Leaf, Caraway, Birch Sweet/Tar, Cananga, Cam-phor,

Black Currant Seed, Calamus Root, Blood Orange, Cade, Cajenut,

Buchu, etc. The aromatic oils come in many scents and flavors and are

utilized to heal the body and
mind.

Blood Orange is botanic Citrus Sinensis oil extracted through cold press

procedures from the crude fruit peels of plants. The oils derived from

Italy. Citrus is a fruit tree, which producing spiny evergreen barks with

edible fruits, such as lemon, orange, grapefruit, lime, and pomelo. The

trees from Italy have huge, white flowers, which is where the fra-grance of

Blood Orange arrives. The oils are a deep orange color, which is used as a

therapeutic remedy. Blood Orange oils include agents, such as

antidepressants. In addition, the oil is used as an antiseptic, aphrodisiac,

anti-spasmodic, cordial, nerve stimulant, carminative, deodorant, and as a

tonic circulatory and cardiac healer. The flavors are medium,
which the

oils blend with clary sage, lavender, nutmeg, clove, spicy oils,
lemon,

myrrh, and cinnamon. The oils have a soothing citrus aroma,
which gives

you a tangy fruit expression. Blood Orange oils are sometimes
called

Maltese Orange. The oils derived from origin came from India.
The

French lands, and Italy people continue to use the fragrances. The
Spain

natives use Blood Orange, yet it is called NARANJA. It is recommended

that while using Blood Orange that you avoid sun ex-
posure.

Bergamot's variant Citrus Bergamia, better known as Bergaptene
Free

oils was extracted through cold press procedures from crude
fruit peels.

The plants originated in Italy. The tree has flowers shaped in the
form of

stars, and the leaves are smooth. The tree bears fruit, which resemble

grapefruit and/or oranges, yet the fruits are shaped like
pears.

Bergamot oils is utilized to treat depression, nervousness, stress, hysteria,

fear, anorexia, eczema, psoriasis, and various skin infections. Bergamot

oils blend with jasmine, Rosemary, frankincense, black pepper, Ylang

oils, sandalwood, orange, geranium, cypress, Vetiver, cypress, Mandarin,

etc. Bergamot oils were named after the city of Bergamo, located in

Lombardy. The oils were extended to Italy, Europe, Ivory Coast, Algeria,

Tunisia, as well as Morocco. Avoid using the oils if you have been

exposed to sunlight, which has caused sensitive
skin.

Betel Leaf oils is botanic Piper Betle oil, which was extracted through a

steam distillation process from plant leaves. The oils originated in India.

The twine vine trees are a sister to the pepper family. The oils produce

antiseptic phenol. Due to the richness of starches, tannin, and sugar the

trees are used as a stimulation aid. The oils deliver aids in warming the

mind and body. In addition the oils are used as aphrodisiacs, antiseptics,

carminative, etc. Betel Leaf has medicinal agents, which

strengthen the

gums, enhance teeth life, and freshens, the
breath.

The oils blend with cardamom, lavender, Rosemary, tea tree, eucalyptus,

etc.

Carrot Seed oils is botanic DAUCUS CAROTA. The oils were extracted

through the steam distillation process, which comes from plant
seeds. The

oils derived from France, and are an herbal scent. The deep,
yellowish

colors present Carrot Seed as an excellent skin care solution for
toning

and revitalizing the flesh. The oils are essential oils, which help to
mature
the skin. The oils will freshen and firm the skin. In addition, the
oils assist

in eliminating toxins. You can use Carrot Seed oils to reduce
water

buildup. Furthermore, carrot seed oils work as a detoxifying
agent, which

cleans the liver, body, and digestion system respectively. The oils
relieve

gouty symptoms, arthritis, rheumatism, edema, and works as an
anti-

inflammatory agent. The oils are said to strengthen mucus mem-
branes,

which is at the nose, lungs, and throat area. Influenza and bron-chitis

symptoms may also fade while using carrot seed essential oils. The

extracted oils in the aromatherapy linage can provide you com-fort, hope,

strength and power to continue
life.

Extracted Oils in Aromatherapy

Aromatherapy is extracted oils, which derive from Australia, Egypt,

France, as well as other lands. The oils are intended to serve as a healing

agent, which you can find a wide assortment of essential oils on-line.

Aromatherapy oils are used as a homeopathy healer. The oils principle is

that poison in smaller doses can serve as a healer. Homeopathy is a

medicinal remedy, which assists in healing. The remedies are utilized in

treating acute illnesses, as well as chronic illnesses. In other words, it is a

prevention strategy.

The oils have been used down through the centuries and in mod-ern times

as well. The Hippocrates is known as the father of medicines, which noted that those in good health could benefit from the oils to fight

diseases. Homeopathy remedies came into focus in the later 1700s. A

German physician named Samuel Hahnemann decided that aromatherapy

oils could be used in medical practice as a healer. The doctor decided that

vegetables, natural sources from animals, and minerals when prepared

could aid in healing. Today, the oils are used worldwide, including

throughout the lands of Great Britain, America, and the European

countries. India, Brazil, Australia, etc, all used aromatherapy oils for

centuries and are still using them
today.

How can I learn about the types of essential
oils?

Online you will find various articles, which will inform you of

aromatherapy's history, the types of oils available, etc. For instance,

Curry Leaf is aromatherapy's essential oils, which its botanic name is

Murraya Koenigi. The oil was extracted from plant leaves through a

steam process. Curry Leaf derived from India, and extracted from the

curry trees. The curry tree is a bushy tree, which grows throughout the

lands of India. The tree produces pale yellowish leaves. Currently

however, Curry Leaf has no available documentation to support its

common use. However, Curry Leaf has been utilized to fight against hair

loss, diabetes, and as an agent to restore skin pigmentation. The oils are

available in medium scents or flavors, as well as strong scents. The oils

are sweet and spicy with a touch of bitter-
ness.

Cypress Australian Blue is an essential oil. The oils botanic name is

known as Callitris Intra-tropica. The oils were extracted from the needles

and twigs of plants and processed via steam. Cypress derived from

Australia, and was extracted from Australia's tropical Cypress trees.

Cypress is a conifer of evergreen trees, which grow through the native

lands of Eurasia, North America, etc, and is made up of hardwoods and

dark green leaves. The leaves resemble scales. Cypress trees are also

called Cupressus. Cypress oils are commonly utilized to treat skin

conditions, etc. The oils can be used to smooth and moisturize the skin. In

addition, Cypress has been utilized to relax the mind, while acting as a

sedative. You can find cypress oils in medium flavors. The oils will blend

with Lemon Tea Tree and Myrtle Lemon scents. AS well, the oils will

blend with Lavender oils, Geranium, Pine, Sandalwood, Juniper, Jasmine,

Rose, Marjoram, Mandarin, Clary Sage, Orange scents,
etc.

Coffee oils are used to promote awareness, or alertness. The aromas are

similar to fresh brewed coffee. Coffee oils work best as stand-alone's. The

oils are utilized as a deodorizer, which the scents are burnt. Coffee oils

act as an antioxidant, aiding to fight depression, nausea, fevers,

respiratory   problems,   and   bee
stings.
Chilly Seed is an essential oil, which derived from Mexico. The oils

botanic name is Capsicum Annum. The oils were extracted from plant

seeds through a steam distillation process. The oils are utilized as an

analgesic, which works as an anti-inflammatory agent, as well as a

digestive system supporter.
Relax with Aromatherapy

Aromatherapy is scented oils or essential oils, which people burn, use as

décors, etc. The oils are claimed to have healing agents, which come from

natural sources. Most oils are extracted from plants, brushes, trees, etc.

The natural agents assist in soothing the body and mind, helping both to

relax. Essential oils and scented oils have been utilized for thousands of

years by foreign members. Egyptians used the oils in massage and

medicinal therapy, which the people in the lands also used the oils as an

embalmment.

Down through the years many others from France areas found use of

aromatherapy as well. Each decade passing brought forth new ideas when

newfound discoveries came into focus. The oils has been tested on and

off for centuries. Today, aromatherapy is used as well as a healing

remedy. Still, few medical doctors will recommend the use of scented oils

to heal the body and mind. The oils come in mild, medium, and strong

scents. Few oils work as standalones to aid in healing, while other oils

blend with various scented oils to enhance
healing.

The stronger oils are idea for those with chronic condition. The
mild and

medium oils work best for those relieving minor symptoms,
stress, etc.

Aromatherapy oils have its own design and works in various ways
to aid

in healing the body and mind from an assortment of health related

problems. Emotional and mental well-being is the resolve
claimed of

scented and essential oils. That is, the oils claim to heal the emotions and

mental responses, so that the body can function
well.

How do I choose aromatherapy
oils?
Knowing what the oils can do is the start to deciding which oils
will work

best for you. What do you want the oils to accomplish? Are you
searching

for oils that spark romance? Do you want oils that heal? Having an
idea

of what your intentions are is a great start to finding aromatherapy oils

best suited for you. Having an overall idea of what types of oils
are

available can also help you make a
choice.

Few of the oils available include Cumin Essential Oils. The oils
botanic

name is Cuminum Cyminum. The oils were extracted by the use
of steam

from plant seeds, which derived from Egypt. Cumin oils are medium

scents, which is used as antiseptics, anti-oxidants, anti-spasmodic, as well

as antitoxic. The oils work as an aphrodisiac to set romantic
moods as

well. In addition, the oils work to fight bactericidal, depurative,

carminative, digestive problems, etc. You can use Cumin oils to
relieve

osteoarthritis symptoms, muscular pain, bloating, indigestion,
headaches,

nervous exhaustion, migraines,
etc.

You can purchase Cumin oils in mild or medium scents, which the
oils

blend with Chamomile, Angelica Root, Rosemary, Oriental Flavors,

Lavender, and Caraway oils.

Another of aromatherapy oils is Cypress French oils, which is an
essential

oil. The botanic oils known as Cupressus Sempervirens were extracted by

steam from the needles and twigs of plants. Cypress originated from

Australia and is used to fight varicose
veins.

In addition, Cypress French oils are utilized to relieve hemorrhoids, feet

perspiration, oily skin, menorrhagia, rheumatism, etc. The oils also aid in

skin care and relieving stress. Cypress French oils blend with Lemon
scents, Juniper, Orange scents, Pine, Tangerine, Rosemary, Lavender,

Juniper, etc. According to Legends, the stake in which Jesus Christ was

annihilated on was made of Cypress Wood, which is a representa-
tion of

death.

Additional oils available to you is the Cinnamon Bark and Leaf, Citral,

Clary Sage, Citronella and Java Citronella, Clementine, Coffee, Clove

Bud and Leaf, Cognac, Cypress Australian Blue, Curry Leaf, Copaiba

Balsam, Cumin, Coriander, Curcuma, etc. Now we can learn a few more

details related to aromatherapy.

Aromatherapy Details

According to reviews the market is saturated with a variety of Cedarwood

oils, as well as Atlas oil. Many of the Cedarwood oils assist in relieving

cellulite, acne, bronchitis, arthritis, anxiety, catarrh, dandruff, eczema,

cystitis, greasy skin, fungal infections, dermatitis, rheumatism, ulcers,

stress, skin irritations, hair loss, etc. Cedarwood Himalayan is an essential

oil, which offers the highest caliber in promoting spiritual needs.

Black Currant Seed is an essential oil, which its Latin name is RIBES

NIGRUM. The oils were extracted via a cold press procedure from the

seeds of plants. The root of this oil comes from the United States of

America. Black Currant is a small dried grape, which the seedless grape

originally came from the Mediterranean areas. The oils are used in

cooking. The small plants grow fruits shrubs. The deciduous shrubs are

cultivated in temperate areas, and are sometimes called RIBES. Black

Currant oils are used to treat linoleic acids, reducing prostoglands, and

correct deficiency in acid production. The results of its action works to

increase blood flow, reduce clotting and inflammation: As well the oils

aid by fighting diabetes mellitus, multiple sclerosis, atherosclerosis,

eczema, PMS symptoms, and so on. Black Currant is also an additive in

particular cosmetics and skin care products. Black Currant blends with

vanilla, Rosemary, jasmine, rosewood, palmarosa, lavender, rose,

eucalyptus, tea tree, lime and lemon. As well, black currant seed oils will

blend with bergamot. Black Currant is sometimes known as Quinsy

Berry.

Birch Tar oils has a Latin name known as Betula Alba. The oils are

extracted from bark, and are processed through steam distillation. Birch
Tar oils origin is Japan. The trees are tall trees with peeling barks and

they grow in the northern hemisphere. The thin, paper, peeling barks

produce dark brown limbs. The oils are commonly used as an ointment.

The ointment works to treat psoriasis, a variety of skin infections,

eczema, etc. You can also use the oils to fight off mosquitoes.

Pharmaceutical remedies are available that include Birch Tar oils, which

the remedies are used to treat dermatological illnesses. The medium scent

oil blends with Rosemary, Jasmine, Cananga, sandalwood, and Benzoin.

Birch Sweet oils Latin name is Betula Lenta. The oils are extracted from

plant bark, which is processed through steam distillation. The origin of

Birch Sweet is Russia. Birch Sweet is a taller tree with peeling bark as

well. The trees grow in the Northern regions. As well Birch Sweet grows

in Southeastern America, southern regions of Canada, and currently the

trees are grown in Eastern Europe, as well as Russia.

The oils produced are clear in color. Birch Sweet oils are essential oils

used as anti-inflammatory agents, analgesic, anti-pryetic, antiseptic, etc.

The oil has proven to efficiently work as massaging oil, which relieves

sprains, sore muscles, aching joints, etc. The strong scent blends with

copaiba, Cedarwood, sandalwood, spruce, rosewood, fir balsam, Peru balsam, pormouwood, etc. The oil produces a sweet, mint scent.

Camphor is another of aromatherapy's essential oils. The oil was extracted through steam distillation process. The oil comes from plant wood, and processed from root stump, chipped woods, branches, etc. China is Camphor's origin, which the chemical-based compound has an antiseptic property. The strong smell is used in medical creams, which relieves itching. IN addition, the plant wood is used to make plastic, celluloid, and explosives. Camphor is utilized as an anti-inflammatory agent, antiseptic, etc. The oils work to by treating cardiac problems, diuretic, carminative, or colic, febrifuge, laxative, etc. Camphor is also used as an insecticide, stimulant, etc. The oil helps relieve nervousness, depression, inflammation, aches and pains, arthritis, acne, bronchitis, colds, flu, fevers, coughs, etc. The strong scented oil blends with Pennyroyal, Chamomile, Cajuput, Basil, Melissa, Rosemary, and lavender. Caraway oils blend with Camphor as well. Camphor was utilized to fight Persia plagues. IN addition, Iran or Persia used Camphor as an embalmer. China utilized the wood to build a variety of their

property. Choosing aromatherapy requires research.
Choosing Aromatherapy

Choosing aromatherapy is sometimes difficult, since there is a wide

assortment available on the market with each doing its own duty. One of

the choice oils is Ocimum Basilicum. The sweet basil oils are other

choice aromatherapy treatments available. The oils deliver a spicy aroma,

which is similar according to reviews, to pasta sauce. The oils aroma is

distinct that vendors have decided to classify the oils, listing them for its

aromatic scents.

In other words, the oils are set apart from the botanic aromatherapy oils.

The fresh smells deliver a light spicy fruit aroma with a twist of balsamic.

Anise scents is an undertone of these oils. The oils aid by giving those

who smell the scents a warming feeling. In addition, the oils tone your

mood, while restoring your peace of mind. The oils aid in fighting

depression. In addition, these oils uplift, clarify, and energize your body

and mind.

The oils blend with clary sage, lavender, bergamot, thyme, cedar wood,

hyssop oils, and geranium oils. The oils will clear your mind, as well as

relieve symptoms of fatigue. The oils are utilized for external use, and are

recommended to be diluted before applying to your skin. Basil oils is

utilized to relieve bronchitis, aches and pains, colds, pains from

childbirth, congestion, fatigue, head colds, depression, hysteria, insect

bites, herpes, headaches, flu, etc. In addition, basil oils work by

enhancing awareness, concentration, confidence, etc. You can use basil

oils to fight indigestion, insomnia, PMS symptoms, mental exhaustion,

migraines, nausea, physical and mental fatigue, stress, nervousness,

rheumatism, shingles, sinus problems, aching muscles, etc. Basil also

assists in reducing indecisiveness by promoting, or stimulating your

mental. You can use basil oils to fight negative thoughts, sorrow, and

stimulate the adrenaline. The oils reduce stress by uplifting your

emotional, mental, and physical being.

Bergamot is one of the choice aromatherapy oils available online. The

botanic Latin name for bergamot is Citrus Bergamia. The oils were

extracted through a cold press process, which comes from crude fruit

peels. The plants originated in
Italy.

Bergamot is a spiny Asian citrus tree. The tree bears sour fruits in the

shape of pears. Oils coming from the bergamot tree are a yellow-ish green

fragrance along the essential oil line, which the oils are extracted from the

rinds of the fruit. Bergamot is also used to make perfumes. In addition,

bergamot is akin to the Mediterranean mint plants. The plants source is

similar to bergamot oils, which its Latin name is Mentha Citrata.

Bergamot oils are commonly used to treat depression, anxiety, stress,

hysteria, fear, and a variety of skin infections. In addition, ber-gamot oils

will treat psoriasis, anorexia, eczema, etc. Bergamot blends with clary

sage, black pepper, frankincense, jasmine, cypress, Rosemary,

Ylang oils,

geranium, Mandarin, sandalwood, Nutmeg, and Vetiver oils.

Bergamot oils deliver a citrus scent, which is warming and sweet to the

smell. Bergamot has an agent in it however that can cause harsh burns,

especially if the oils are applied to sensitive skin.

Cedarwood Himalayan is an aromatherapy essential oil. Its Latin name is

Cedarus Deodora. Cedarwood Himalayan was extracted through a steam distillation process, which the oils come from wood. The wood is found

in the Himalayas located in India.

The oil is made in a pale yellowish color, which the oil is used as an

antiseptic. In addition, Cedarwood is used as an ant putrescent, etc. This

oil is also used as an aphrodisiac, anti-seborrheic, astringent, fungicidal,

etc. IT seems this oil combines to aid in a variety of health issues, and

mental issues respectively. In addition, the oils are used to set off

romantic moods. The strong aroma blends with citrus oils, Rosemary, eucalyptus, and chamomile oils. Aromatherapy is a therapeutic way to

heal the body and mind.

Healing the Body and Mind with Aromatherapy

Aromatherapy comprises essential and scented oils. The oils are designed

to help relieve stress. As well, the oils are used to heal the body and mind

of ailments, which the fragrances work to relieve pressure while healing

the soul.

Aromatherapy's essential oils are oils made from natural trees, roots,

plants, etc. The oils are intended to reinstate or preserve overall health.

The essential oils come in a variety of fragrances. Aromatherapy oils

work to offer serene to the body, while pampering the soul. The body and

mind will feel refreshed according to claims after using particular

aromatherapy oils. Aromatherapy is a treatment scheme made of plant

oils, which are extracted from plants and intended to alleviate

psychological and physical disorders. The oils are used as inhalants or

massage therapy. In addition, you can use aromatherapy oils as décors,

fresheners, etc.

Cassia is one of aromatherapy's essential oils. The oils botanic name is

pronounced as CINNAMOMUM Cassia. The oils were extracted via a

steam method, which came from plant leaves. The oil originates in

Vietnam. Cassia is a tree, which its bark is scented with evergreen. The

Asian tree's aromatic bark aids in the production of Cassia oils. The name

CINNAMOMUM Cassia is a Latin based name. Cassia is dark brown oil,

which is commonly used as a tonic, stimulant, and/or carminative.

Carminative helps to relieve flatulence symptoms, such as colic. The oils

expel gas from the alimentary canal. As well, Cassia oils are used as an

aid for nausea, diarrhea, etc. The oils were studied by Japan and China

labs, which results showed that Cassia could also be used as a sedative, as

well as treating high blood pressure. The oils also reduce fevers, and

works as an antiseptic. In addition, Cassia oil can fight fungi, bacteria,

rheumatism, colds, arthritis, fevers, influenza, etc. The strong scents work

well with Ginger, Benzoin, and Frankincense, Coriander, Grapefruit,

Cloves, Thyme, Rosemary, and Lavender oils. Cassia oils are also
called

the "Bastard Cinnamon" as well China Cinnamon. Cassia was used
in

China for thousands of years as a medicine. The first known use of
Cassia

was in A.D. 200, or 200 B.D. This was at the time of Han Dynasty.
The

oil has side effects, which include irritability to the mucus membrane.

Dermal sensitizer and dermal irritability is another side effect. In

addition, it is recommended that pregnant women avoid using
Cassia oils.

Basil essential oils are another of aromatherapy's line, which
pregnant

women should also avoid. Basil's botanic name is OCIMUM

BASLICUM, which derives from Latin. The oil was extracted
through

steam distillation from the leaves and flowers of plants. Basil originated

in Italy, yet the oils have been used in various areas. Basil is an
aromatic

plant, sometimes known as an herb, Rosemary, Sage, Thyme, or
Parsley.

Basil oils are used to strengthen empathy yet it is also used as a
sinus

reliever. Basil is sometimes used to heal digestive problems, as well as

stimulate the circulation system. IN addition, basil is used to heal

respiratory complications. The strong aroma blends with Clary Sage,

Juniper, Clove Bud, Eucalyptus, Bergamot, Rosemary, Lemon, Lime, and

Neroli. Basil is titled the Royal Remedy by the Greeks. Sometimes the

Greek call Basil the King. Indians, Mediterranean areas, and Asia all

adore this aromatherapy solution.

Online you can find a wide assortment of aromatherapy oils. The oils

include Blood Orange, Coffee, Bergamot, Chilly Seed, Carrot Seed, Celery Seed, Cinnamon Leaf and Cinnamon Bark, etc. IN the same areas

you will find a short history available to you, which you can use to select

the best aromatherapy treatment.
Aromatherapy Healing You

Aromatherapy has been well-though out down through the century as a

remedy that soothes the mind and body. The preparations are claimed to mitigate symptoms coming from an assortment of mental and physical

illnesses. In addition, the remedies are claimed to reduce stress, anxiety,

nervous tension, as well as related symptoms. Many people down through

the years have utilized aromatherapy, including the French natives,

Egyptians, Germans, Brazilians, Europeans, Indians, Canadians,

Americans, people in the Mediterranean lands, and so on. The oils

include the scented and essential oils. Online you can find a variety of the

oils, including Basil, Cedarwood, celery seed, carrot seed, African

Bluegrass oils, bergamot, clove bud and leaf oils, and so on. The oils each

have its intention for therapeutically healing the body and mind. Before

employing aromatherapy oils be, sure to read all available instructions.

Some of the oils may include side effects.

How do I choose aromatherapy oils?

Everyone is different. Making your choice depends on you and what you

are seeking to accomplish. You can ask a few questions to help you make

a decision.

Questions:

Do I want aromatherapy oils to ignite romance?

Can I benefit from using aromatherapy as a stress reliever?

Do I have any mental or physical illnesses, which aromatherapy could

read relieve my symptoms?

Are my intentions to freshen my car or
home?

Can I use aromatherapy scents and fragrances as a
décor?
What about perfumes?

As you can see aromatherapy is used in a variety of ways. It is up
to you

what you want to use the oils for, however if you answered yes to
any or

all of the questions above you may want to consider Bergamot,
Basil,

Jasmine, and so on.

If you are considering aromatherapy for décor purposes, you may
want to

combine oils with the selection of jars and bottles. In the aromatic line

you will find glass bottles, plastic jars, Boston shape bottles, steel

canisters, acrylic jars, and so on. You can find a variety of caps and
tops

as well. Amber bottles are ideal to compliment aroma therapeutic oils.

You can find dealers online as well who will customize the bottles and

jars to your liking. You will find a variety of sizes, colors; designs
etc in

the bottle and jar line as well. The colors range from Cobalt blue,
amber,

clear colors, frosted jars, dark greens, black, etc. Unique, modern
and

funky designs are also available.

If you're looking for little romance, i.e. to spark romance tryout
jasmines

line, as well as bergamot. Bergamot works as a body and mind
healer as

well, which it includes an apha-
siac.

Soap additives, soap, and botanical extracts, as well as fragrance
and

essential oils are available as well. The soaps or additives are
highly

recommended moisturizing formulas, and are not artificially
colored. The

products have been tested on animals, and incorporate hundred
percent

vegetable made. As well the products are biodegradable, non-
yellowing,

and are superb clarities.

You can find a nice line of clear products, bathe butter foams, goat milk,

white, liquid crystalline and liquid organic concentrated products, liquid

suspending crystal, organic, olive, shea butter, soy, SLS free oils, and

more online.

Benzoin essential oils are commonly used as an antiseptic, anti-

inflammatory agent, antidepressant, deodorant, colic and related

symptoms reliever, etc. Benzoin is also used as a perfume. The oils aid in

treating coughing, colds, bronchitis, acne, wounds, scar tissue, psoriasis,

eczema, arthritis, rheumatism, mouth ulcers, muscle pain, etc. You can

use the oils as a circulation activator, stress reliever, to reduce tension,

and so on. A selection of other aromatherapy oils and products are

available to you for the taken, yet it is up to you to make the right choice

as to what oils are best suited for your needs. In all aromatherapy is a

healing solution.

Aromatherapy the Healing Solutions

Cyproil is one of the essential oils available online that works as an aromatherapy solution. The botanic oils known as Cyperus Scarious were

extracted through a steam process from flowers. The Brazilian oil is a

grassy plant, which has floral scented and delicate flowers. The oils are

dark amber and sometimes light brown. Cyproil is commonly used in

compounds perfumes, soaps, incense, and medicine. You can also use the

oil as an insect repellent. The natural smelling oils blend with patchouli,

bergamot, labdanum, and clary sage.

Cypress French oils, sometimes called Cupressus Semperiviren. The oils

come from needles and twig from plants, and are extracted through a

steam process. The Australian oils are pale yellowish, and are commonly

used to fight foot perspiration, menorrhagia, hemorrhoids, rheumatism,

varicose veins, oily skin, and has worked to relax the mind and body. The

oil is also used to relax the nerves and treat the skin with its astringent

property. The medium scent oils work with Fennel oils, bergamot,

grapefruit oils, lime, lemon, Rosemary, orange, Juniper, clary sage,

lavender, pine, and so on. Tangerine oils work blend well with cypress

French oils. According to legends Cypress oils derives from the same

wood used as a stake in Jesus Christ's mur-
der.

Cypress Australian Blue is an essential oil, named Callitris Intrat-
ropica

also. The oil comes from needles and twigs, and is extracted via a steam

process. The oil originated from Australia, which the trees are family to

the Southern Conifer. The beautiful blue oils are commonly used to treat

skin by soothing and moisturizing the flesh. Aroma therapists use this oil

as an agent to sooth and relax the nerves without sedating the pa-
tient. The
medium strength oils blend with lavender oils, Cedarwood oils, Lemon

Tea Tree, Pine oils, Lemon Myrtle, orange, geranium oils, clary sage,

rose oils, mandarin, cardamom, jasmine oils, sandalwood oils, juniper,

marjoram oils, and so on.

Curry Leaf oils are along the essential oil line. The botanic oils named

Murraya Koenigi are extracted via steam and come from plant leaves.

The India based oil comes from diminutive bushes from India, which the

bushes grow in the Himalayas, Burma, and throughout the eastern areas.

The oils are pale yellow, and are used by the India natives as a culinary

remedy. However, there is no available information to claim what curry

leaf oil does to heal the body and
mind.

Curcuma essential oils come from the Latin name Curcuma Aromaticum.

The plant seeds were steam extracted, and the origin of the plants is India.

Curcuma is a tropical plant, which comes from turmeric, zeodoary, and is

extracted as aromatherapy oils. The oils are yellow or yellowish green.

Curcuma is commonly used to relax and balance the nerves. The oil has

an antiseptic application, as well as agents to heal the skin, including

acne. It is claimed that this oil will reduce growth of female facial hair.

The medium aroma blends with spicy blends, ginger, Ylang oils, Clary

Sage, etc.

Cumin essential oils derive from the Latin name Cuminum Cyminum.

The oils are extracted via steam and come from plant seeds. Egypt is the

origin of this oil. The oils are found in various parts of the Mediterranean

areas. The cumin plants grow aromatic
seeds.
The Mediterranean plants are a member of the carrot family and it grows

small pink and white flowers. The flowers are grown for the specific

purpose of extracting its aromatic seeds. However, the seeds are

sometimes used as spice in cooking. The common use of the oils treat a

variety of symptoms, including muscle pain, osteoarthritis, bloating,

nervous tension, headaches, digestive problems, dyspepsia, colic, and so

on. The oils have antiseptics, aphrodisiacs, anti-toxics, antispasmodic,

bactericidal, and so on. The oil will also treat migraines. The medium

strength aroma blends with Oriental flavors, essential oils, lavender,

chamomile, caraway, Rosemary, Angelica Root, and so on. A variety of

all aromatherapy oils are available online.

A Variety of Aromatherapy Oils

Costus root's Latin name is Sassuriea Costus. The oils were ex-tracted

from plant roots and processed via steam. The India based oils grow

black flowers, which the dried plant roots are separated, soft-ened, and

soaked in warm water. The plants are then made into Costus root through

the steam distillation process. The oils are brown or yellow, and the

common use is to work as an antiseptic, antiviral, febrifuge,

antispasmodic, bactericidal, and so on. The oils are claimed to heal those

dealing with hypertension, stomach acids, and so on. In addition, Costus

root oils is used to make perfumes and cosmetics. Costus roots are also an

ingredient in Soda pops and alcohol, as well as in specific foods. The soft

aromas blend with Ylang oils, floral scents, patchouli, Oriental oils, and

so on. Costus Root however is a dermal irritant, which is not

recommended as an aromather-apy.

Coriander essential oils also named Corriandrum Sativum was extracted

via the steam distillation process from plant seeds. The Russia based oil

produces aroma from its plant. The plants are from the native lands of

Asia and throughout Mediterranean areas, and are grown for the purpose

of its aromatic leaves. The aroma is also used in cooking. The oils are

also called Chinese parsley. Coriander oils are clear or pale yellow and

are commonly used as an aphrodisiac, analgesic, deodorant,

antispasmodic, and so on. The oils relieve mental fatigue, rheumatism,

nervous disorders, tension, migraines, arthritis, colds, flu, muscle spasms,

and so on. The medium strength aromas blend with cinnamon, orange,

pink or white oils, ginger, lemon, and so on. The people through-out the

lands of Egypt used Coriander more so as an aphrodisiac. India used the
oils as a flavoring for foods, while the Greeks and Romans used the oils

to flavor their wine.

Copaiba Balsam is another of the essential oils known as Copaif-era

Officinalis. The oils were steam distilled extracted from crude resin

plants. Copaiba Balsam begun in Brazil, yet the oils are now spread throughout the country. The pale yellow oils are commonly used to

balance, soothe and uplift the mind and body. Blended aroma-therapy oils

used with Copaiba Balsam is said to extend life. The medium strength

oils blend with spicy oils, floral oils, etc. The oil also has an aphro-disiac

agent, which works well with Jasmine, sandalwood, rose, frankin-cense,

vanilla, Ylang oils, and so on. The oils are also used in colognes, soap,

perfumes, detergents, and so on.

Clove Bud oils named Syzgium Aromaticum as well, came from India.

The oils were extracted via steam distillation methods from plant buds.

The aromatic spices present a strong aromatic scent, which were distilled

from the dried flower buds of the tropical clove trees and used as a

flavoring for sweet and spicy foods. The evergreen trees come from the

family of myrtle, and from native Moluccas. In addition, the buds are

grown in various tropical regions. The light golden yellow oils are

commonly used as a treatment for mild aches and pains, such as tooth aches, etc. The oils will help fight colds and flu as well. The scents come

in both medium and strong and blend with spicy oils, peppermint,

grapefruit, Citronella, Rosemary, rose, orange oils, and lemon oils.

Clementine is an essential oil sometimes known as Citrus Nobilis. The

oils were extracted from crude plant peels and through a cold press

procedure. The plant originated in Italy. The pale yellow oils are commonly used to revitalize the soul, whilst balancing sleep. Insomniacs

could benefit from using this oil. The medium strength oil blends with

floral and citrus family scents.

Aromatherapy Blends

Botanic oils include Salvia Sclarea, otherwise known as Clary Sage. The

oil was extracted via a steam distillation process, extracted from plant

flowers and leaves. The Bulgaria based plants are herbs with hairy-like

leaves, and are large in form. The oils extracted from the plants are light

golden yellow. The oil is commonly used as an aromatherapy, including

used as an antidepressant, sedative, antispasmodic, tonic, deodorant,

hypertension healer, and so on. The oil has also been known to assist in

relieving asthma symptoms and spasms. The medium or strong scented

oil blends with a variety of essential oils, including German, bergamot,

Roman, chamomile, Cedarwood, Neroli, jasmine, rosewood, lavender,

orange, geranium, sandalwood, Ylang oils, and so
on.

Citronella Java oils also called Cymbopogon Winterianus comes from the

gum plants and is steam distilled, extracted from the plants. The

beginning of citronella arrives at Sri Lanka. The lemon aromatic grass is

an Asian tropical bluish green, lemon aromatic leave, and contains

aromatic oils. The oils are used in perfumes, and are used as an insect

repellent. The oils are yellowish brown, and are used as an aromatherapy.

The oils include antiseptics, insecticide, deodorant, tonics, and parasitic.

Used with Cedarwood flavors the oil can work well as an insect repellent.

The oils are also used to make candles, soaps, etc. You can use the oils to

fight flu and cols, as well as oily hair/skin and perspiration. The medium

scents blend with in variety of oils, including pine, bergamot, lavender,

bitter orange, orange, Cedarwood, lemon, and Geranium oils. Still, it is a,

predominate insect repel-
lent.
Another of the botanic oils available is the Citral essentials. The oil was

extracted via the steam distill process, which came from stems and roots

from plants. China is the beginning, yet China is far from the end of this

oils roots. The oils are light yellow and commonly used as an antiseptic,

invigorator, antidepressant, and works to heal the nerves, and soothe pain

and aches. The oil produces a strong lemon scent, as well as an

herbaceous scent. The oils will treat athletic foot odors and itching, acne,

scabies, oily skin, and will help to reduce
stress.

The botanic aromatherapy Chilly Seed oils were distilled from steam and

plant seeds. The Mexico based oils also comes from plants in Southern

America and Central America. The rich, reddish orange oils are

commonly used in aromatherapy, since it has an analgesic agent, anti-inflammatory agent, and an aid to the digestive system. The strong scents

do not blend with other oils.

When you are searching for aromatherapy oils it is best to shop online.

Shopping online gives you advantages, including live support. In other

words, you can find Live Chat Support online to help you find oils that

may not be listed in the series of articles. I thought I would throw this in

to give you a briefing on how shopping online can bring you a variety of

benefits.

Continuing Chenopodium essential oils were extracted from plant fruit

and leaves and distilled through the use of steam. The Russia based oils

are commonly used in a variety of problems. The oils will work to

remove roundworms, Ascaride, as well as treat diuretics. The strong scent

does not blend with other oils. The oils are sometime called the American

Wormseed Oils.

Choulmogra is another of the essential oils utilized in treating

rheumatism, skin disease, eczema, scrofula, bruising, sores, sprains,

leprosy, and so on. The oil derived from India but is currently utilized all

over the world. For additional information on aromatherapy and
essential

oils go online where you will find a variety of helpful information.

aromatherapy also has a line of extracts.